CYCLING EXERCISE FOR SENIORS OVER 60

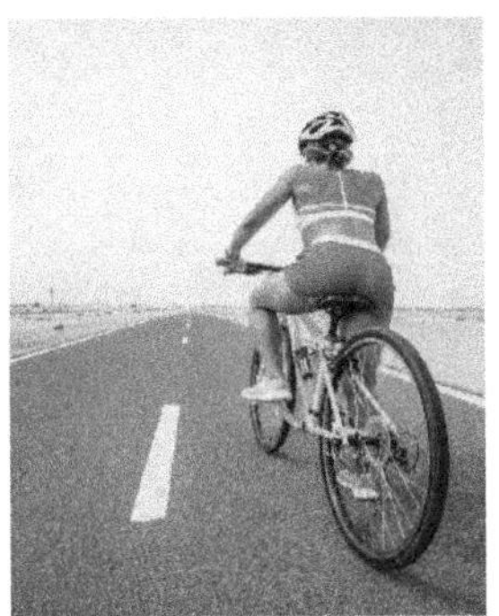

A Comprehensive Guide to Overcoming Challenges, Embracing Joy, and Fostering Well-Being Through the World of Cycling.

By

Michelle T. Rills

Table of contents

About the Book

Cycling for Seniors: A Guide to Active Aging" is an indispensable resource designed to empower individuals over 60 to embrace the numerous physical and mental benefits of cycling. The book begins with a compelling introduction, emphasizing the importance and advantages of incorporating cycling into the lives of seniors. It sheds light on the transformative impact of this exercise on overall health and well-being.

Addressing health considerations is a pivotal aspect of the guide, stressing the necessity of consulting healthcare providers and implementing safety precautions. Readers will find detailed insights into selecting the right bike, understanding the various types suitable for seniors, and ensuring proper sizing for comfort and efficiency.

Essential gear and accessories are explored, emphasizing the significance of protective gear and suitable clothing. The guide doesn't merely focus on physical aspects; it delves into warm-up routines and stretching exercises tailored to seniors, promoting flexibility and joint health.

Structured workout plans are outlined, emphasizing frequency, duration, and gradual progression to accommodate different fitness levels. Safety on the road is a key concern, with dedicated sections on traffic awareness and riding in varied conditions.

Readers are guided through the social dimensions of cycling, encouraging participation in group activities and community events. Common concerns, such as joint health and fatigue, are addressed with practical advice.

The book distinguishes itself by incorporating real-life case studies and success stories, providing inspiration and relatable experiences. It concludes with an extensive FAQ section, anticipating and answering common queries about senior cycling. "Cycling for Seniors" serves as a comprehensive guide, offering not only practical tips but also fostering a sense of community and motivation for seniors embarking on this enriching journey.

Introduction

Embarking on the golden years doesn't mean slowing down; instead, it's an opportunity for active aging and embracing the numerous benefits of cycling. In this comprehensive guide, 'Cycling for Seniors: A Guide to Active Aging,' we delve into the transformative power of cycling as a means to enhance physical fitness, mental well-being, and overall quality of life for individuals over 60.

The introduction sets the stage by highlighting the profound importance of incorporating cycling into the lives of seniors, emphasizing that this is not just an exercise but a lifestyle that fosters vitality and longevity. It underlines the multifaceted advantages, ranging from cardiovascular health and joint flexibility to the positive impact on mental acuity and mood.

The book navigates through the initial considerations, urging seniors to consult healthcare providers and follow safety precautions, ensuring a holistic approach to well-being. A critical aspect is the exploration of the diverse types of bikes suitable for seniors and guidance on selecting the right one, coupled with insights on proper sizing for comfort and efficiency.

Beyond the physical, the guide addresses the significance of warm-up routines and tailored stretching exercises designed to promote flexibility and joint health. Structured workout plans cater to various fitness levels, emphasizing a gradual progression to make cycling accessible to everyone.

As we unfold the pages of this guide, readers will discover the joy of cycling as a social activity, fostering a sense of community through group activities and participation in events. Real-life case studies and success stories add a personal touch, providing inspiration and relatability.

In essence, 'Cycling for Seniors' is not merely a guide; it is an invitation to a vibrant and fulfilling chapter of life, where the road ahead is paved with health, happiness, and the invigorating breeze of the open trail."

Foreword

In the quiet town of Silver Springs, where time seemed to slow down, a group of spirited seniors found themselves on an unexpected journey—one that would redefine their golden years. It all began with a weathered book nestled on the community center's shelf, its title catching the eye of a curious soul: 'Cycling for Seniors: A Guide to Active Aging.'

As they cracked open the pages, the quaint town transformed into a haven of spinning wheels and open trails. The introduction of the guide echoed through the town square, awakening a desire for active living among its seasoned residents. The once hushed streets now echoed with laughter and the gentle hum of bicycle wheels.

The book became a beacon, illuminating the path to a lifestyle that transcended the limitations often associated with aging. It wasn't just about exercise; it was about embracing the freedom of movement and the wind in one's hair. The seniors gathered in the community center, exchanging stories of their youthful cycling adventures and dreams of rediscovering that joy.

Guided by the wisdom of the book, they explored health considerations, consulted with local healthcare providers, and adorned themselves with helmets and vibrant cycling jerseys. The town soon witnessed a colorful parade of bikes, each carefully selected for comfort and style, as the seniors discovered the perfect fit.

The story unfolded through warm-up sessions in the town square, group rides along scenic paths, and shared moments of triumph and camaraderie. The guide not only provided practical advice on structured workouts but also became a source of inspiration through real-life tales of individuals who had pedaled their way to renewed vigor.

As the wheels turned, Silver Springs transformed into a vibrant community, a testament to the power of 'Cycling for Seniors.' The introduction to this book marked not just the beginning of a new chapter but an unfolding adventure of health, friendship, and the timeless joy of the open road."

Chapter 1

1.1 Importance of Cycling for Seniors

For seniors, cycling is very important since it provides a variety of social, mental, and physical benefits that enhance overall wellbeing.

1. Cardiovascular Health: By strengthening the heart and promoting blood circulation, frequent cycling helps to promote cardiovascular health. Consequently, this lowers the chance of developing heart disease and keeps blood pressure within a safe range.

2. Joint Flexibility and Strength: Cycling is a great low-impact activity for seniors because it's easy on the joints. It increases muscle strength, encourages joint flexibility, and helps to preserve bone density, all of which improve mobility overall.

3. Weight Management: Cycling turns into a useful technique for weight management as metabolism slows down with age. In addition

to assisting with weight maintenance and calorie burning, it lowers the incidence of obesity-related illnesses.

4. Mental Well-Being: Riding a bike provides advantages for mental health in addition to its physical health. Endorphins, or "feel-good" hormones, are released, which lessen stress, anxiety, and depressive symptoms. Cycling's rhythmic quality can have a meditative effect, encouraging calmness and relaxation of the mind.

5. Balance and coordination: Cycling improves these abilities, which are critical for reducing falls, a problem that many seniors have. Combining various motor abilities is necessary for the exercise, which increases stability all around.

6. Social Engagement: Seniors who ride bikes have a great opportunity to maintain their social lives. Cycling organizations, community activities, and group rides all help to create a supportive community by

fostering a sense of togetherness and lowering social isolation.

7. Independence and Freedom: Seniors who ride bikes have a sense of freedom and independence. They can have an active and satisfying existence by using their bike to explore their surroundings, run errands, and enjoy the outdoors.

Cycling is an important and fun exercise for those navigating their golden years because, in essence, its significance goes beyond physical fitness and involves a holistic approach to health, emotional well-being, and social connection.

1.2 Benefits of Cycling for Individuals Over 60

For people over 60, riding a bicycle has many advantages that improve their overall quality of life, mental and physical health, and overall physical health.

1. Cardiovascular Fitness: Cycling regularly strengthens the heart and circulatory system and promotes cardiovascular health. It promotes a better cardiovascular profile by lowering the risk of high blood pressure, heart disease, and stroke.
2. Joint Health and Low Impact: Cycling is a low-impact exercise, making it gentle on the joints. It provides an effective way to improve joint flexibility, reduce stiffness, and alleviate arthritis symptoms without placing excessive strain on the knees and hips.
3. Muscle Strength and Endurance: Pedaling engages various muscle groups, including the legs, thighs, and core. This helps build and maintain muscle strength, improving overall endurance and supporting daily activities.

4. Weight Management:As metabolism tends to slow with age, cycling becomes a valuable tool for managing weight. Regular cycling helps burn calories, maintain a healthy weight, and reduce the risk of obesity-related conditions.

5. Improved Balance and Coordination: Cycling requires a coordinated effort between various muscle groups, contributing to improved balance and coordination. This is particularly beneficial for seniors in preventing falls and maintaining stability.

6. Cognitive Benefits: Engaging in physical activity like cycling has positive effects on cognitive function. It can help maintain mental acuity, reduce the risk of cognitive decline, and contribute to better overall brain health.

7. Mood Enhancement: Cycling stimulates the release of endorphins, the body's natural mood elevators. This leads to reduced stress, anxiety, and symptoms of depression, fostering a positive mental state.

8. Social Interaction: Participating in group rides, cycling clubs, or community events provides opportunities for social interaction. This social engagement contributes to emotional well-being, reduces feelings of isolation, and fosters a sense of community.

9. Independence and Freedom: Cycling offers a sense of independence and freedom for individuals over 60. It enables them to explore their surroundings, run errands, and enjoy outdoor activities, contributing to an active and fulfilling lifestyle.

In conclusion, cycling is a comprehensive exercise that benefits seniors' physical and mental well-being as well as their social connections. Because of its many advantages, people navigating the opportunities and challenges of their elderly years often find it to be a fun and approachable exercise.

Chapter 2

Health Considerations

2.1 Consultation with Healthcare Provider

Consultation with a healthcare provider is a crucial step before embarking on a cycling regimen, especially for individuals over 60. Here are key reasons why seeking professional advice is essential:

1. Health Assessment:
A healthcare provider can assess an individual's overall health, taking into account pre-existing medical conditions, medications, and any potential contraindications. This evaluation forms the basis for creating a personalized cycling plan that aligns with the individual's health needs.

2. Addressing Existing Conditions:
Seniors may have specific health concerns or chronic conditions that require consideration. Consulting with a healthcare provider allows for tailored recommendations, ensuring that cycling

activities are safe and beneficial, taking into account conditions such as arthritis, heart disease, or respiratory issues.

3. Medication Considerations:
Some medications may impact a person's ability to engage in certain physical activities. Healthcare professionals can review medications and provide guidance on how cycling might interact with these drugs, ensuring safety and minimizing potential risks.

4. Individualized Exercise Prescription:
Healthcare providers can prescribe an exercise plan that aligns with an individual's fitness level, health goals, and any restrictions they may have. This personalized approach maximizes the benefits of cycling while minimizing the risk of injury or exacerbation of health issues.

5. Safety Precautions:
Seniors may have specific safety considerations related to their health status. Healthcare providers can offer advice on injury prevention, proper warm-up routines, and guidelines for gradually increasing exercise intensity to avoid strain or overexertion.

6. Monitoring Progress:
Regular check-ins with a healthcare provider allow for the monitoring of progress and adjustments to the exercise plan as needed. This ongoing dialogue ensures that the cycling routine remains effective and safe, adapting to any changes in the individual's health.

In summary, consultation with a healthcare provider serves as a foundational step for seniors considering cycling. It provides a comprehensive understanding of an individual's health status, allowing for the development of a tailored and safe exercise plan that promotes overall well-being.

2.2 Safety Precautions

It is crucial to ensure riding safety, especially for those who are older than 60. The following are crucial safety measures to adhere to:

1. Health Check-Up: See a doctor before beginning a riding regimen to determine whether cycling is

appropriate for your specific condition and to evaluate your general health.

2. Appropriate Bike Fit: To enhance comfort and lower the chance of strain or injury, make sure your bike is the right size and fitted to your body. Seek expert guidance as necessary.

3. Protective Gear:
Always wear a well-fitted helmet to protect your head in case of falls or accidents. Consider additional protective gear such as knee and elbow pads for extra safety.

4. Visibility:
Wear brightly colored or reflective clothing, especially during low-light conditions. Equip your bike with lights and reflectors to enhance visibility to motorists and pedestrians.

5. Warm-up Exercises:
Engage in warm-up exercises to prepare your muscles and joints before cycling. This helps prevent injuries and enhances flexibility.

6. Gradual Progression:

Start with shorter rides and gradually increase the duration and intensity of your cycling sessions. This allows your body to adapt and reduces the risk of overexertion.

7. Safe Routes:
Choose cycling routes that are well-maintained, have clear signage, and avoid heavy traffic when possible. Familiarize yourself with local bike paths and trails.

8. Regular Maintenance:
Regularly inspect and maintain your bike. Check brakes, tires, and gears to ensure they are in good working condition. Promptly address any mechanical issues.

9. Hydration:
Stay well-hydrated, especially during longer rides. Carry water with you and take regular breaks to prevent dehydration.

10. Weather Awareness:
Be mindful of weather conditions. Adjust your cycling plans based on factors such as rain, wind, or

extreme temperatures. Dress appropriately for the weather.

11. Emergency Preparedness:
Carry a fully charged mobile phone, identification, and any necessary medications. Familiarize yourself with basic first aid procedures and emergency contact information.

12. Road Rules:
Obey traffic rules and regulations. Use hand signals to indicate turns, and be predictable in your movements. Stay alert to your surroundings.

13. Group Cycling Precautions:
If cycling in a group, communicate effectively and maintain a safe distance from other cyclists. Be aware of the group's pace and adjust accordingly.

People over 60 who prioritize these safety measures can reap the rewards of cycling—both psychologically and physically—while lowering the risks that may arise from this fulfilling pastime.

Chapter 3
Choosing the Right Bike
3.1 Types of Bikes for Seniors

For seniors, selecting the correct kind of bike is essential to comfort and usability. The following are a few bike types that are appropriate for those over 60:

1. Comfort Bikes:

Designed for a relaxed riding position, comfort bikes feature a comfortable saddle, easy gearing, and an upright handlebar. They are ideal for casual rides on smooth surfaces.

2. Step-Through Bikes (Low-Step Bikes):

These bikes have a low or no top tube, making it easy to mount and dismount. Step-through bikes are especially suitable for seniors with limited mobility or those who prefer the convenience of easy access.

3. Cruiser Bikes:

Known for their laid-back design, cruiser bikes offer a comfortable, upright riding position. They are great for leisurely rides on flat terrain and often come with wide, cushioned saddles.

4. Electric Bikes (E-Bikes):

E-bikes come with an electric motor to assist pedaling. This can be beneficial for seniors who may need a boost on inclines or for longer rides. E-bikes offer various levels of pedal assistance.

5. Recumbent Bikes:
With a reclined seating position, recumbent bikes reduce strain on the back and neck. They are a good option for seniors with back issues or those looking for a more relaxed riding experience.

6. Three-Wheeled Bikes (Trikes):
Trikes provide stability with three wheels, making them a safe choice for seniors concerned about balance. They often feature a comfortable seat and a basket, making them practical for errands.

7. Hybrid Bikes:
Combining features of road and mountain bikes, hybrids offer versatility. They typically have a comfortable riding position, wide tires, and are suitable for both paved and light off-road trails.

8. Folding Bikes:
Folding bikes are compact and easy to store, making them convenient for seniors with limited space.

They are also practical for combining cycling with other modes of transportation.

9. Adult Tricycles:

Similar to trikes, adult tricycles provide stability with three wheels. They often have a comfortable, wide seat and are suitable for leisurely rides or errands around the neighborhood.

10. Road Bikes with Flat Handlebars:

For seniors who prefer a more traditional cycling experience, road bikes with flat handlebars provide a streamlined design with a slightly upright riding position.

It's important to take comfort, individual preferences, and any physical limits into account while selecting a bike. Seniors can discover the ideal bike for their needs and have a safe and happy cycling experience with the assistance of test rides and consultations at a nearby bike store.

3.2 Proper Bike Sizing

For seniors in particular, the right bike sizing is essential to a productive and comfortable riding experience. To guarantee the proper bike size, keep the following points in mind:

1. Standover Height: Ensure there's adequate clearance between the top tube and your inseam when straddling the bike with your feet flat on the ground. For road bikes, a clearance of 1-2 inches is recommended, while mountain bikes may allow for more clearance.

2. Frame Size: The frame size is a fundamental factor. Consult the manufacturer's size chart or seek assistance from a bike shop to determine the appropriate frame size based on your height and leg length.

3. Reach and Handlebar Height: The reach to the handlebars should be comfortable, allowing a slight bend in your elbows when holding the grips. Adjust the handlebar height to ensure a relaxed, not overly leaned-forward, riding position.

4. Saddle Height: Set the saddle height to achieve a slight bend in your knee when the pedal is at its lowest point in the pedal stroke. A proper saddle height promotes efficient pedaling and reduces the risk of knee strain.

5. Saddle Position: Adjust the saddle forward or backward to find the optimal position for your riding style. This helps in achieving a balanced and comfortable posture.

6. Handlebar Width: Ensure the handlebar width matches your shoulder width. This promotes better control and a more natural riding position.

7. Stem Length: The stem length influences your reach to the handlebars. Choose a stem length that complements your upper body proportions, providing a comfortable and controlled grip.

8. Crank Arm Length: The length of the crank arms affects the pedal stroke. Consider

shorter crank arms for comfort and reduced strain, especially if you have joint issues.

9. Test Rides: Whenever possible, take the bike for a test ride before purchasing. This allows you to assess comfort, handling, and any adjustments needed for your specific preferences.

10. Professional Assistance: Seek advice from a bike shop professional or a bike fitting specialist. They can provide personalized guidance based on your body measurements and riding style.

Seniors may ensure that their bike fits properly and provides a comfortable and joyful cycling experience while also promoting overall safety and well-being by considering these components of correct bike fitting.

Chapter 4

Essential Gear and Accessories

4.1 Helmets and Protective Gear

Seniors riding must use protective gear, including helmets, to ensure their safety. Below is a summary of essential protective gear:

1. Helmet:

Fit: Choose a helmet that fits snugly on your head, level and covering your forehead. It should not be too tight or too loose.

Straps: Adjust the straps so they form a V-shape under your ears, with the buckle centered beneath your chin. Tighten the straps enough to prevent movement but not to the point of discomfort.

2. Eye Protection:

Sunglasses or Clear Lenses: Protect your eyes from wind, debris, and UV rays. Choose glasses with UV protection for sunny days or clear lenses for low-light conditions.

3. Gloves:
Padding: Cycling gloves provide padding to absorb vibrations and protect your hands during long rides. Grip: They offer a better grip on the handlebars and protect your palms in case of a fall.

4. Knee and Elbow Pads:
Protection: Especially relevant for mountain biking or if you're prone to falls, these pads provide an extra layer of protection for your joints.

5. Reflective Clothing:
Visibility: Wear clothing with reflective elements, especially if cycling in low-light conditions. This enhances visibility to motorists and other cyclists.

6. Bright and Reflective Outerwear:
Visibility: Consider a bright and reflective jacket or vest for added visibility, especially when riding in the early morning or late evening.

7. Proper Footwear:
Closed-toe Shoes: Wear closed-toe shoes with good traction to ensure a firm grip on the pedals. Consider cycling-specific shoes for enhanced performance.

8. Arm Warmers and Leg Warmers:
Temperature Regulation: In cooler weather, these accessories help regulate your body temperature while providing an extra layer of protection.

9. Hi-Vis Accessories:
Accessories: Attach reflective accessories, such as ankle bands or clip-on lights, to enhance visibility from various angles.

10. Padded Shorts:
Comfort: Padded shorts provide extra cushioning, reducing discomfort during longer rides.

Keep in mind that using protective gear correctly determines its efficiency. Check your equipment frequently for indications of wear and tear, and replace any necessary parts. In the end, getting high-quality safety equipment makes riding a bike safer and more pleasurable—especially for older riders.

4.2 Comfortable Clothing and Footwear

Choosing comfortable clothing and footwear is crucial for an enjoyable and safe cycling experience, especially for seniors. Here are some considerations:

1. Moisture-Wicking Clothing:

Opt for moisture-wicking fabrics that draw sweat away from your body. This helps keep you dry and comfortable during rides.

2. Padded Shorts:

Consider wearing padded shorts for extra comfort, especially during longer rides. The padding helps reduce friction and provides cushioning.

3. Breathable Fabrics:

Choose clothing made from breathable materials to enhance airflow and regulate body temperature.

4. Layering for Temperature Control:

Dress in layers, especially in cooler weather. This allows you to adjust your clothing as needed to maintain a comfortable temperature.

5. Bright and Visible Colors:

Wear bright and visible colors to enhance your visibility to others on the road. This is particularly important for safety, especially in low-light conditions.

6. Close-Fitting Sleeves:

Opt for close-fitting sleeves to prevent any interference with the bike's moving parts and to reduce wind resistance.

7. Comfortable Shoes:

Wear closed-toe shoes with good arch support. Cycling-specific shoes with stiff soles can enhance pedaling efficiency.

8. Non-Slip Grip Gloves:

Use non-slip grip gloves to enhance your grip on the handlebars. This is particularly helpful during hot or rainy weather.

9. Reflective Accessories:

Incorporate reflective accessories, such as ankle bands or reflective strips on your clothing, to improve visibility to others, especially during low-light conditions.

10. Adjustable Clothing:
Choose clothing with adjustable features like waistbands or cuffs, allowing you to customize the fit for maximum comfort.

11. Sun Protection:
Wear sun-protective clothing or apply sunscreen to exposed skin to guard against harmful UV rays.

12. Helmet-Friendly Hairstyles:
Opt for hairstyles that fit comfortably under your helmet, avoiding any discomfort or interference.

By paying attention to these clothing and footwear considerations, seniors can ensure a comfortable and enjoyable cycling experience. It's essential to prioritize comfort and safety when selecting gear to make the most of each ride.

Chapter 5

Warm-up and Stretching Exercises

5.1 Importance of Warm-up

It is impossible to emphasise the value of warm-ups before beginning any workout programme, especially one that involves cycling for seniors. Warm-ups are important for the following main reasons:

1. Increased Blood Flow:

Warming up gradually increases blood flow to your muscles, delivering oxygen and nutrients. This prepares your body for the increased demand during exercise, reducing the risk of injury.

2. Improved Muscle Elasticity:

Gentle warm-up activities, such as light aerobic exercises or dynamic stretches, improve muscle elasticity. This enhances the range of motion in joints, making movements smoother and reducing the likelihood of strains or sprains.

3. Raised Body Temperature:
Warm-ups elevate your body temperature, which is beneficial for optimal muscle function. Warmer muscles contract and relax more efficiently, improving overall muscle performance.

4. Joint Lubrication:
As you warm up, synovial fluid production increases, lubricating the joints. This helps reduce friction between joint surfaces, enhancing joint flexibility and reducing the risk of injuries like tendinitis.

5. Mental Preparation:
Warming up provides a mental transition from rest to activity. It allows you to focus on your workout, enhances concentration, and prepares you for the physical demands of cycling.

6. Activation of Nervous System:
A proper warm-up activates the nervous system, promoting better communication between your brain and muscles. This coordination is crucial for balance, stability, and efficient movement.

7. Injury Prevention:

By gradually preparing your body for more intense activity, warm-ups significantly reduce the risk of injuries, particularly strains, pulls, and other muscular or joint-related issues.

8. Enhanced Cardiovascular Function:
Warming up gradually increases your heart rate, preparing your cardiovascular system for the increased demands of cycling. This ensures a smoother transition from rest to exercise and helps prevent sudden stress on the heart.

9. Improved Performance:
A well-executed warm-up primes your body for optimal performance. It allows you to perform at your best, whether you're cycling for leisure, fitness, or more competitive purposes.

10. Faster Recovery:
Warming up may contribute to a faster recovery post-exercise. By gradually easing into activity, your body adapts more efficiently, potentially reducing muscle soreness and stiffness.

For seniors engaging in cycling, where joints and muscles may need extra care, a thoughtful warm-up routine becomes even more critical. It's a proactive approach to ensure a safe, enjoyable, and effective exercise session while promoting overall well-being.

5.2 Specific Stretches for Seniors

Stretching is a crucial component of any exercise routine, providing seniors with benefits such as improved flexibility, joint mobility, and reduced muscle stiffness. Here are some specific stretches tailored for seniors, particularly beneficial before cycling:

1. Neck Stretch:
   - Gently tilt your head to one side, bringing your ear toward your shoulder.
   - Hold for 15-30 seconds, feeling the stretch along the side of your neck.
   - Repeat on the other side.

2. Shoulder Rolls:
   - Lift your shoulders towards your ears in a circular motion.
   - Repeat for 10-15 seconds, then reverse the direction.

3. Wrist Flexor Stretch:
- Extend your arm in front of you with the palm facing down.
- Use your opposite hand to gently press down on the fingers.
- Hold for 15-30 seconds and switch sides.

4. Chest Opener:
- Stand tall, interlace your fingers behind your back, and straighten your arms.
- Lift your arms slightly, opening your chest.
- Hold for 15-30 seconds.

5. Trunk Rotation:
- Sit on a chair with your feet flat on the ground.
- Twist your upper body to one side, holding the back of the chair for support.
- Hold for 15-30 seconds and repeat on the other side.

6. Hip Flexor Stretch:
- Stand with one foot forward and the other foot back.
- Bend your front knee and gently lower your back knee toward the ground.

- Hold for 15-30 seconds and switch sides.

7. Quadriceps Stretch:
- Stand near a sturdy surface for balance.
- Lift one foot toward your buttocks, holding the ankle with your hand.
- Hold for 15-30 seconds and switch legs.

8. Calf Stretch:
- Stand facing a wall with your hands on it.
- Step one foot back, keeping it straight, and press the heel into the floor.
- Hold for 15-30 seconds and switch legs.

9. Ankle Circles:
- Sit comfortably and lift one foot off the ground.
- Rotate your ankle in a circular motion for 10-15 seconds in each direction.
- Switch legs and repeat.

10. Seated Forward Bend:
- Sit on the edge of a chair with your feet flat on the ground.
- Hinge at your hips and reach forward toward your toes.

- Hold for 15-30 seconds, feeling a stretch in your hamstrings and lower back.

The main muscle groups that these stretches are intended to target are those that increase mobility and flexibility. Never forget to move slowly and deliberately while doing each stretch—avoid making jerky or abrupt motions. Before beginning a new stretching regimen, it is advisable to speak with a healthcare provider if you have any current health issues.

Chapter 6

Structuring Cycling Workouts

6.1 Frequency and Duration

The frequency and duration of stretching exercises for seniors can vary based on individual fitness levels, health conditions, and personal preferences. However, a general guideline for incorporating stretching into a routine is as follows:

Frequency:

- Aim for at least 2-3 days a week to include stretching exercises in your routine.
- Ideally, perform stretches on days when you are not engaging in more intense physical activities like cycling or strength training.

Duration:

- Hold each stretch for 15-30 seconds. This duration allows your muscles and connective tissues to lengthen gradually without causing strain.

- Repeat each stretch 2-4 times, depending on your comfort level.

Additional Tips:
- Prioritize consistency over intensity. Regular, gentle stretching yields better results than occasional, intense sessions.
- Listen to your body. If a stretch feels uncomfortable or causes pain, ease off and adjust the intensity.
- Include a variety of stretches to target different muscle groups and improve overall flexibility.

For seniors engaged in cycling, incorporating stretching into the routine becomes particularly important to enhance joint mobility and reduce muscle stiffness. A well-rounded approach, combining cycling, stretching, and potentially strength training, contributes to overall physical well-being.

6.2 Gradual Progression

A fundamental component of any fitness programme is gradual growth, which is particularly crucial for seniors, who may include cyclists in their regimen. Here's why it's important to move gradually and how to do so:

1. Injury Prevention: Progressing gradually reduces the risk of injuries. Sudden increases in exercise intensity or duration can strain muscles and joints, especially for seniors who may have age-related considerations.

2. Adaptation: Your body needs time to adapt to new physical activities. Gradual progression allows your muscles, joints, and cardiovascular system to adjust, leading to improved endurance and strength over time.

3. Joint Health: Seniors often have considerations related to joint health. Gradual progression helps the joints adapt to increased demands, reducing the risk of overuse or strain.

4. Cardiovascular Adaptation: For activities like cycling, gradual progression ensures that your cardiovascular system can adapt to the increased demands on your heart and lungs. This supports better endurance and overall cardiovascular health.

5. Sustainable Habits: Gradual progression supports the development of sustainable habits. Consistency is key in maintaining an active lifestyle, and a gradual approach helps avoid burnout or frustration.

How to Progress Gradually:
1. Start with Short Sessions: Begin with shorter cycling sessions, especially if you're just starting or returning to regular exercise. Aim for a duration that feels comfortable, then gradually increase over time.

2. Increase Intensity Slowly: If you're incorporating more challenging routes or higher resistance on a stationary bike, do so gradually. Allow your body to adapt to the increased effort.

3. Add Variety: Introduce variety into your cycling routine by incorporating different terrains or cycling styles. This can include intervals of increased speed or resistance.

4. Listen to Your Body: Pay attention to how your body responds to each session. If you experience persistent discomfort or fatigue, consider scaling back and progressing more slowly.

5. Monitor Recovery: Ensure you have adequate time for recovery between sessions. Recovery is when your body strengthens and adapts to the demands of exercise.

6. Regular Assessments: Periodically assess your fitness level and adjust your cycling routine accordingly. This could include increasing duration, intensity, or incorporating new challenges.

7. Include Rest Days: Plan regular rest days to allow your body to recover. Rest is an

essential component of any fitness routine and aids in preventing overtraining.

Seniors can reap the benefits of cycling while lowering their risk of injury and guaranteeing a fun and sustainable workout regimen by using a progressive progression method. Before beginning a new fitness programme, always get medical advice, especially if you have any underlying health issues.

Chapter 7

Safety Tips on the Road

7.1 Traffic Awareness

Traffic awareness is crucial for cyclists, especially seniors, to ensure a safe and enjoyable riding experience. Here are key tips for maintaining awareness and safety while cycling in traffic:

1. Obey Traffic Laws:

Follow the same traffic rules as motorists. Obey traffic signals, stop signs, and road markings to enhance predictability for yourself and other road users.

2. Be Visible:

Wear bright and reflective clothing to enhance visibility, especially in low-light conditions. Use lights on your bike during dawn, dusk, or night rides.

3. Use Hand Signals:

Indicate your intentions to motorists by using clear and recognizable hand signals for turning or stopping. This helps drivers anticipate your movements.

4. Be Predictable:

Ride in a straight line, and avoid sudden maneuvers. Being predictable makes it easier for motorists to anticipate your actions.

5. Stay Alert:

Keep your eyes on the road, scanning for potential hazards. Stay aware of the traffic around you, including vehicles, pedestrians, and other cyclists.

6. Make Eye Contact:

Attempt to make eye contact with drivers at intersections or when crossing paths. This ensures that they see you and are aware of your presence.

7. Choose Safe Routes:

Plan your route to include roads with designated bike lanes or lower traffic volume. Familiarize yourself with cycling infrastructure in your area.

8. Check Blind Spots:

Be aware of motorists' blind spots, especially around larger vehicles. Ensure you are visible and avoid lingering in blind spots.

9. Maintain a Safe Distance:
Keep a safe distance from parked cars to avoid opening doors. Similarly, leave ample space between yourself and moving vehicles.

10. Listen for Traffic:
Use your hearing to be aware of oncoming traffic, especially if riding in areas with limited visibility.

11. Be Mindful of Weather Conditions:
Adjust your cycling plans based on weather conditions. Rain, snow, or fog can impact visibility and road conditions.

12. Anticipate Intersections:
Approach intersections cautiously, even if you have the right of way. Be prepared for potential conflicts with turning vehicles.

13. Respect Pedestrians:
Yield to pedestrians in crosswalks and be considerate when sharing paths with walkers.

14. Know Your Surroundings:

Be familiar with the road layout and potential hazards on your route. This awareness helps you navigate confidently and safely.

By incorporating these traffic awareness tips into your cycling routine, seniors can enjoy the benefits of cycling while minimizing risks associated with sharing the road with other vehicles. Always prioritize safety and stay vigilant while cycling in varied traffic conditions.

7.2 Riding in Varied Conditions

For seniors in particular, riding in a variety of situations can be gratifying and hard. The following advice can help you ride safely and enjoyably in a variety of conditions:

1. Adjust to the Weather:

Be ready for varying weather conditions. When dressing for the weather, take into account waterproof clothing. Keep yourself hydrated and shield yourself from the sun during hot weather.

2. Choose Appropriate Routes:
Select routes that match your comfort level and riding ability. Some paths may be better suited for certain weather conditions or offer more shelter from wind

3. Adjust Riding Style in Wind:
In windy conditions, ride with a lower profile by bending your elbows and tucking in. This reduces wind resistance and makes cycling more comfortable.

4. Mind Road Surfaces:
Different surfaces, such as asphalt, gravel, or dirt, can affect your ride. Adjust your speed and technique accordingly, and be cautious of potential hazards like potholes.

5. Handle Wet Surfaces:
Wet roads can be slippery. Reduce your speed, avoid sudden maneuvers, and be cautious when turning or braking. Use fenders to minimize water splashes.

6. Stay Visible in Low Light:

In low-light conditions or at dusk, wear reflective clothing and use lights on your bike to enhance visibility. Make sure your front and rear lights are in good working order.

7. Check Tire Pressure:

Adjust tire pressure based on the conditions. Lower pressure can provide better traction on softer surfaces, while higher pressure is suitable for smoother roads.

8. Mind Temperature Extremes:

In extreme heat, stay hydrated and plan rides for cooler parts of the day. In cold weather, layer clothing to stay warm and protect against wind chill.

9. Plan for Steep Hills:

If your route includes steep hills, adjust your gear accordingly. Use lower gears for easier climbs and higher gears for descents. Practice proper braking technique on descents.

10. Carry Essentials:

Pack essentials like water, a small toolkit, and a map or GPS device. Ensure your mobile phone is charged in case you need assistance.

11. Ride in Groups:

Riding with a group can enhance safety, especially in challenging conditions. Group members can provide assistance and support if needed.

12. Be Mindful of Traffic:

In busy or congested areas, stay alert and be mindful of traffic patterns. Signal your intentions clearly and use hand signals when necessary.

13. Regular Bike Maintenance:

Ensure your bike is well-maintained, especially if you frequently ride in varied conditions. Check brakes, tires, and gears regularly.

By adapting your approach to different conditions and staying prepared, seniors can continue to enjoy the benefits of cycling in diverse environments. Always prioritize safety, be aware of your surroundings, and make adjustments to your riding style as needed.

Chapter 8

Group Cycling and Social Benefits

8.1 Joining Cycling Clubs

One of the best ways for seniors to improve their cycling experience is to join a group. Here are some advantages and pointers for cycling club membership:

Advantages:

1. Social Interaction: Seniors can interact with like-minded people who share their passion for cycling in the social setting that cycling clubs offer.

2. Attend Introductory Events: A lot of groups provide rides that are suitable for beginners or introductory events. Attend these to meet other members and get a sense of the club's dynamics.

3. Think about Club Culture: Every club has a distinct purpose and culture. Some people might value social rides more than competition. Select a club based on your aims and preferences.

4. Ask About Rides That Are Senior-Friendly: Find out whether there are any rides that are slower-paced or designed especially for senior citizens. There are groups in certain clubs that are especially designed to accommodate different ability levels.

5. Verify Membership Conditions: Recognise the prerequisites for membership, including any costs and the anticipated level of dedication. Certain clubs might let guests ride specific rides or offer trial memberships.

6. Safety Measures: Give clubs that prioritize safety on rides top priority. This entails following traffic laws, using appropriate signals, and coordinating with one another.

7. Ask About Riding Schedules: Find out if the club's riding schedule coincides with your

free time. Certain clubs provide rides on certain weekdays, weekends, or evenings.

8. Participate and Contribute: Take an active role in club events and show a willingness to make a constructive contribution to the team. This promotes a feeling of camaraderie among club members.

In addition to improving your riding experience, joining a bicycle club can give you support and a sense of community. It's a great way for seniors to keep active, inspired, and in touch with other cyclists who share their passion.

8.2 Community Events and Rides

Participating in community events and rides can add a vibrant and social dimension to a senior's cycling routine. Here are some benefits and tips for joining community events and rides:

Advantages :

1. Social Engagement: Community events and rides offer opportunities to connect with other cyclists and members of your community. It's a chance to share experiences and build friendships.

2. Motivation and Inspiration: Being part of a larger cycling event can be motivating. The collective energy and enthusiasm can inspire you to challenge yourself and set new goals.

3. Variety of Routes: Community events often feature diverse routes that showcase the beauty of the local area. This allows you to explore new paths and enjoy different landscapes.

4. Inclusivity: Many community rides are designed to be inclusive, catering to cyclists of various skill levels. This makes them accessible for seniors who may prefer a more relaxed pace.

5. Support and Safety: Larger events typically have support services, including route marshals, aid stations, and medical

assistance. This enhances safety and provides a sense of security.

6. Sense of Accomplishment: Completing a community ride, especially if it's a more extended or challenging route, can provide a great sense of accomplishment and boost your confidence in your cycling abilities.

Tips for Participating:

1. Research Local Events: Look for local cycling events or rides in your community. Check online platforms, community bulletin boards, or visit local bike shops for information.

2. Choose Events Wisely: Consider your fitness level and preferences when choosing events. Some may be more leisurely, while others may focus on longer distances or challenging terrains.

3. Prepare and Train: If the event involves longer distances or more challenging routes, ensure you're adequately prepared. Gradually

increase your training to build the stamina required for the event.

4. Register Early: Many community events have limited spaces, so consider registering early to secure your spot. This also gives you ample time to prepare and plan.

5. Connect with Event Organizers: Reach out to event organizers if you have specific questions or concerns. They can provide valuable information about the route, support services, and any special considerations for seniors.

6. Bring a Friend: Consider participating with a friend or fellow cyclist. It adds to the enjoyment and provides mutual support during the event.

7. Check Equipment: Ensure your bike is in good condition before the event. Check the tires, brakes, and gears to avoid any technical issues during the ride.

8. Stay Hydrated and Fueled:

Bring water and snacks to stay hydrated and energized during the ride. Many events provide aid stations, but it's wise to have your own supplies as well.

9. Enjoy the Experience:
Participate with a positive mindset, focusing on the enjoyment of the ride and the camaraderie of fellow cyclists.

Joining community events and rides can inject excitement and a sense of community into your cycling routine. It's an opportunity to celebrate your love for cycling alongside others who share the same passion.

Chapter 9

Post-Ride Recovery

9.1Cooling Down Exercises

Cooling down after cycling is essential for promoting recovery, flexibility, and reducing muscle soreness. Here are some cooling down exercises for seniors after a cycling session:

1. Gentle Cycling:
- Finish your ride with a few minutes of gentle, easy-paced cycling. This helps gradually decrease your heart rate and eases the transition from exercise to rest.

2. Quadriceps Stretch:
- Stand with one hand against a stable surface for support.
- Bend your knee, bringing your heel toward your buttocks, and hold your ankle with your hand.
- Feel the stretch in the front of your thigh.
- Hold for 15-30 seconds and switch legs.

3. Hamstring Stretch:

- Sit on the edge of a chair or bench with one leg extended straight in front of you.
- Hinge at your hips and reach toward your toes.
- Feel the stretch along the back of your thigh.
- Hold for 15-30 seconds and switch legs.

4. Calf Stretch:

- Stand facing a wall and place your hands against it.
- Step one foot back, keeping it straight, and press the heel into the ground.
- Feel the stretch in your calf.
- Hold for 15-30 seconds and switch legs.

5. Seated Forward Bend:

- Sit on the floor with your legs extended straight in front of you.
- Hinge at your hips and reach toward your toes.
- Feel the stretch in your hamstrings and lower back.
- Hold for 15-30 seconds.

6. Hip Flexor Stretch:
- Kneel on one knee with the other foot in front, forming a 90-degree angle.
- Shift your weight forward, feeling a stretch in the front of your hip.
- Hold for 15-30 seconds and switch sides.

7. Chest Opener:
- Stand tall and clasp your hands behind your back.
- Lift your arms slightly, opening your chest.
- Hold for 15-30 seconds, focusing on stretching your chest and shoulders.

8. Neck and Shoulder Rolls:
- Gently roll your shoulders backward and forward.
- Drop your ear to one shoulder, feeling a stretch on the opposite side of your neck.
- Repeat on the other side.

9. Ankle Circles:
- While seated, lift one foot off the ground and rotate your ankle in a circular motion.
- Repeat for 10-15 seconds in each direction.
- Switch legs and repeat.

10. Deep Breathing:

- Finish your cooling down routine with deep, slow breaths. Inhale deeply through your nose, hold for a moment, and exhale slowly through your mouth.

Do not forget to take your time and be careful when completing these exercises for cooling down. As you pay attention to your breathing, let your pulse rate progressively drop. After your riding ride, cooling down can help with flexibility and muscle healing as well as your general feeling of wellbeing.

9.2 Hydration and Nutrition Tips

Staying properly hydrated and maintaining good nutrition are crucial for seniors engaged in cycling. Here are some tips to help you stay hydrated and nourished during and after your rides:

Hydration Tips:

1. Drink Water Regularly:

Sip water throughout your ride, even if you don't feel excessively thirsty. Dehydration can occur gradually, so it's essential to maintain a consistent fluid intake.

2. Hydrate Before Riding:
Drink water before starting your ride to ensure you begin in a well-hydrated state. This sets the foundation for maintaining hydration during cycling.

3. Consider Electrolytes:
For longer rides or in warmer weather, consider beverages with electrolytes to replace salts lost through sweating. Coconut water and sports drinks are examples.

4. Monitor Urine Color:
Check the color of your urine. Light yellow or pale straw usually indicates proper hydration, while dark yellow may suggest dehydration.

5. Hydration During Hot Weather:
In hot weather, increase your fluid intake to compensate for additional fluid loss through sweating. Aim to drink before you feel thirsty.

6. Avoid Excessive Caffeine and Alcohol:

Limit caffeine and alcohol intake as they can contribute to dehydration. Opt for water or hydrating beverages instead.

Nutrition Tips:

1. Pre-Ride Fuel:

Consume a balanced meal or snack 1-2 hours before your ride. Include carbohydrates for energy, protein for muscle support, and a small amount of healthy fats.

2. On-the-Bike Snacks:

Bring easily digestible snacks like energy bars, bananas, or trail mix for rides longer than an hour. These provide a quick energy boost.

3. Post-Ride Recovery:

Eat a balanced meal or snack within an hour of finishing your ride. Include a mix of carbohydrates and protein to replenish energy stores and support muscle recovery.

4. Include Protein:

Ensure your overall diet includes an adequate amount of protein to support muscle maintenance and repair. Good sources include lean meats, dairy, beans, and nuts.

5. Healthy Fats:
Include sources of healthy fats, such as avocados, nuts, and olive oil, in your diet. These contribute to overall health and can provide sustained energy.

6. Fruits and Vegetables:
Aim for a variety of fruits and vegetables to ensure you get a range of vitamins, minerals, and antioxidants. These support overall health and recovery.

7. Stay Balanced:
Strive for a balanced diet that includes a mix of carbohydrates, proteins, fats, vitamins, and minerals. This helps provide sustained energy and supports your overall well-being.

8. Listen to Your Body:
Pay attention to hunger and fullness cues. Eat when you're hungry and stop when you're satisfied. This helps maintain a healthy relationship with food.

Remember, individual nutritional needs can vary, so it's advisable to consult with a healthcare professional or a registered dietitian for personalized advice based on your health status and specific dietary requirements.

Chapter 10

Case Studies and Success Stories

10.1 Real-life Experiences of Seniors Cycling

Seniors' actual experiences in life Cycling is a great way to demonstrate the many mental, social, and physical health advantages it offers. The following recurring themes emerge from the experiences of senior citizens who have taken up cycling:

1. Health and Wellness:
- Better Cardiovascular Health: Regular cycling has been linked to improved cardiovascular health in many seniors. This low-impact workout promotes stronger heart health, more stamina, and better circulation.
- Joint Mobility: Cycling is an accessible workout for seniors because it is easy on the joints. Pedaling lowers stiffness and preserves joint mobility with a flowing action.

- Strength and Balance: Cycling can improve balance and strengthen the legs, which lowers the risk of falls in older adults.

2. Mental and Emotional Benefits:

- Stress Reduction: Seniors often find cycling to be a stress-relieving activity. The rhythmic motion, fresh air, and connection with nature contribute to a sense of calm and well-being.

- Mood Enhancement: Cycling can have mood-enhancing effects. Seniors frequently report feeling a sense of accomplishment, joy, and improved mental clarity after a ride.

- Cognitive Benefits: Regular exercise, including cycling, has been associated with cognitive benefits. Some seniors note improved focus, memory, and overall cognitive function.

3. Social Connection:

- Community Engagement: Joining cycling clubs or participating in community rides provides an avenue for social interaction. Seniors often form friendships, share experiences, and create a sense of community within these groups.

- Shared Activities: Cycling becomes a shared activity for couples or groups of friends. It offers an opportunity to spend quality time together while pursuing a healthy and enjoyable pastime.
- Participation in Events: Seniors often take part in cycling events or charity rides, contributing to a broader sense of community and shared purpose.

4. Independence and Empowerment:
- Increased Independence: Cycling provides a mode of independent transportation for some seniors. It allows them to maintain mobility and access local amenities without relying solely on other modes of transport.
- Empowerment: Seniors who take up cycling often express a sense of empowerment. They challenge stereotypes about aging and demonstrate that an active lifestyle is achievable at any age.

5. Overcoming Challenges:
- Adapting to Physical Changes: Seniors share stories of adapting their cycling routines to accommodate physical changes associated

with aging. This might include choosing different bike styles, adjusting ride intensity, or incorporating rest breaks.

- Overcoming Initial Hesitations: Some seniors initially hesitate to take up cycling due to concerns about balance or stamina. However, many find that starting slowly, seeking support from others, and gradually building up their cycling activities help overcome these initial barriers.

6. Lifelong Learning:

- Learning New Skills: Cycling often involves learning or refining skills, especially if seniors are new to the activity or exploring different types of bikes. This continuous learning process contributes to mental stimulation and a sense of achievement.

These real-life experiences collectively highlight that cycling is more than just a physical activity for seniors; it becomes a holistic lifestyle choice that positively impacts their overall well-being. From improved health to social connections and a sense of empowerment, seniors find diverse and meaningful benefits in embracing cycling.

10.2 Overcoming Challenges

Overcoming obstacles is a crucial aspect of any senior's cycling trip. These are typical problems that seniors encounter along with solutions:

1. Limitations on the body:

*   Challenge: Age-related or health-related physical restrictions may act as a roadblock.
*   Overcoming Strategy: Begin with low-impact activities gradually. To ensure that your riding programme is appropriate for your ability, speak with a healthcare practitioner. Take into account adaptive gear if required.

2. Balance Concerns:

*   Challenge: Seniors may worry about balance, particularly when starting cycling.
*   Overcoming Strategy: Choose a stable bike, such as a tricycle or one with a lower step-through frame. Practice riding in a safe, open

space to build confidence. Consider balance exercises off the bike to improve stability.

3. Safety Apprehensions:
- Challenge: Fear of accidents or injuries can be a significant concern.
- Overcoming Strategy: Invest in safety gear, such as a helmet and reflective clothing. Start with low-traffic areas and gradually progress. Take a cycling safety course if available in your community.

4. Choosing the Right Bike:
- Challenge: Selecting a bike that suits your needs and comfort can be daunting.
- Overcoming Strategy: Visit a local bike shop for expert advice. Test different types of bikes to find one with the right fit and features. Consider comfort and ease of use, such as step-through frames.

5. Motivation and Consistency:
- Challenge: Maintaining motivation and consistency in a cycling routine.
- Overcoming Strategy: Set realistic goals, both short-term and long-term. Find a cycling

buddy or join a club for added motivation. Mix up your routes to keep things interesting. Celebrate your achievements, no matter how small.

6. Weather and Environmental Factors:
- Challenge: Weather conditions or environmental factors can deter seniors from cycling.
- Overcoming Strategy: Check weather forecasts and plane rides on favorable days. Dress appropriately for different weather conditions. Invest in rain gear or use an indoor stationary bike on challenging weather days.

7. Joint Discomfort:
- Challenge: Joint discomfort or arthritis can impact cycling.
- Overcoming Strategy: Choose a bike with a comfortable seating position. Opt for a bike with wider tires for a smoother ride. Consult with a healthcare professional for advice on managing joint discomfort.

8. Transitioning from Inactivity:

- Challenge: Transitioning from a sedentary lifestyle to regular cycling.
- Overcoming Strategy: Start with short, gentle rides and gradually increase duration and intensity. Listen to your body and take breaks as needed. Celebrate progress and focus on the positive impact on your health.

9. Lack of Cycling Knowledge:
- Challenge: Lack of knowledge about cycling etiquette, maintenance, or route planning.
- Overcoming Strategy: Take a cycling workshop or join a local cycling group for guidance. Learn basic maintenance skills or seek assistance from a bike shop. Explore user-friendly cycling apps for route planning.

10. Time Management:
- Challenge: Finding time for cycling within a busy schedule.
- Overcoming Strategy: Schedule cycling sessions like any other appointment. Combine cycling with other activities, such as running errands. Consider shorter, more frequent rides if time is limited.

Overcoming challenges in senior cycling often involves a combination of adapting to individual needs, seeking support, and gradually building skills and confidence. With patience, persistence, and a positive mindset, many seniors successfully integrate cycling into their lives, reaping the numerous physical, mental, and social benefits it offers.

Conclusion

The journey of seniors embracing cycling is a testament to the resilience, adaptability, and determination inherent in this demographic. Overcoming physical limitations, balance concerns, and safety apprehensions, seniors find ways to integrate cycling into their lives, demonstrating that age should not be a barrier to embracing new challenges. The diverse experiences reflect a collective effort to address common challenges, from choosing the right bike to managing joint discomfort.

Motivation and consistency play pivotal roles in sustaining a cycling routine, and seniors often draw inspiration from achievable goals, supportive communities, and the joy of exploration. Realizing that cycling is not just a physical activity but a holistic lifestyle choice, seniors celebrate the mental and emotional benefits that accompany each ride. Social connections, cognitive stimulation, and a sense of empowerment emerge as valuable outcomes, challenging societal stereotypes about aging.

As seniors share their stories of adapting to change, navigating weather conditions, and continuously learning, they inspire others to embark on their cycling journey. The lessons learned in overcoming obstacles extend beyond the bike, fostering a spirit of resilience and an unwavering commitment to a healthy and active lifestyle. In the tapestry of these experiences, seniors illustrate that cycling is not just a means of transportation but a transformative adventure that contributes to their well-being, independence, and the joy of a life well-lived.

Quiz

1. What is a recommended strategy for seniors facing physical limitations in cycling?

a. Start gradually with low-impact activities

b. Jump into intense cycling immediately

c. Choose high-impact activities for quick results

2. What is a common concern for seniors starting cycling related to balance?

a. Fear of riding too fast

b. Fear of accidents or injuries

c. Fear of not enjoying the activity

3. How can seniors overcome safety apprehensions in cycling?

a. Invest in safety gear, such as a helmet and reflective clothing

b. Avoid using safety gear to stay comfortable

c. Ride without considering traffic rules

4. What is a crucial factor when choosing the right bike for seniors?

a. The trendiest bike design

b. The bike's color

c. The right fit and features for comfort

5. What strategy can help seniors maintain motivation and consistency in their cycling routine?

a. Set unrealistic goals

b. Rely solely on willpower

c. Set realistic goals and find a cycling buddy or join a club

6. How can seniors address concerns about joint discomfort while cycling?

a. Ignore joint discomfort for the sake of the ride

b. Choose a bike with a comfortable seating position

c. Stop cycling altogether

7. What can be a common obstacle for seniors transitioning from inactivity to regular cycling?

a. Overexerting in the first ride

b. Starting with short, gentle rides

c. Avoiding breaks during rides

8. Why is lack of cycling knowledge a potential challenge for seniors?

a. It doesn't impact the cycling experience

b. It can lead to unsafe cycling practices

c. Seniors are naturally knowledgeable about cycling

9. How can seniors manage time effectively for cycling within a busy schedule?

a. Scheduling cycling sessions like any other appointment

b. Ignoring time constraints and riding randomly

c. Relying solely on spontaneous rides

10. What role does patience play in overcoming challenges in senior cycling?

a. It is unnecessary

b. It is crucial for sustained progress

c. It hinders progress

11. What can seniors do to address concerns about weather conditions while cycling?

a. Plane rides on favorable days and dress appropriately

b. Avoid cycling altogether during challenging weather

c. Only cycle indoors

12. How can seniors address a lack of motivation to start cycling?

a. Wait for external motivation

b. Set achievable goals and focus on the positive impact

c. Assume cycling won't bring any positive impact

13. What can help seniors build confidence in their cycling abilities, especially regarding balance?

a. Avoiding any cycling until fully confident

b. Practicing riding in a safe, open space

c. Never attempting to ride a bike

14. What is an essential safety consideration for seniors when cycling in traffic?

a. Riding without lights in low-light conditions

b. Using hand signals for turning or stopping

c. Ignoring traffic rules for convenience

15. How can seniors overcome the challenge of transitioning from a sedentary lifestyle to regular cycling?

a. Jumping into long, intense rides immediately

b. Starting with short, gentle rides and gradually increasing

c. Avoiding cycling altogether

16. What is a potential benefit of joining cycling clubs for seniors?

a. Isolation from the community

b. Enhanced social interaction and support

c. No impact on the overall cycling experience

17. What factor is crucial when choosing the right bike for seniors?

a. Trendy bike color

b. Comfort and ease of use

c. The weight of the bike

18. How can seniors address concerns about balance while cycling?

a. Avoid cycling altogether

b. Practice riding in a safe, open space to build confidence

c. Ignore balance concerns and ride anywhere

19. What is a common misconception about starting cycling for seniors?

a. It requires no adaptation or learning

b. It's only suitable for the very fit

c. Cycling has no impact on mental well-being

20. What is a key factor in maintaining motivation for seniors in their cycling routine?

a. Ignoring achievements

b. Celebrating progress, no matter how small

c. Focusing solely on the end goal

Thanks for Reading!!!

A heartfelt thank you to each one of you for taking the time to engage with our content on senior cycling. Your readership, consideration, and support are deeply appreciated. Your interest in exploring the challenges and experiences of seniors embracing cycling adds immense value to our shared knowledge.

Thank you for being a vital part of our community. Your presence and contributions make the journey of learning and discovery all the more meaningful.